PELVIC FLOOR EXERCISES

FOR

WOMEN

Simple Illustrated Workout Guide to Healing Pelvic Prolapses, Incontinences, Pain, Sexual Dysfunctions and Muscle Tightening

DR. SUNSHUN KEVIN

Copyright © 2024 by DR. SUNSHUN KEVIN

All rights reserved.

No part of this publication may be reproduced, distributed or transmitted in any form or by any means, including photocopying, recording, or other electronic or mechanical methods, without the prior written permission of the publisher, except in the case of brief quotations embodied in critical reviews and certain other noncommercial uses permitted by copyright law.

Table of Contents

Introduction

Welcome to the book, "Pelvic Floor Exercises for Women" This book is a comprehensive guide designed to empowe women with knowledge about their pelvic health and provid practical, effective exercises to strengthen the pelvic floor.

A collection of muscles called the pelvic floor creates a kin of hammock across your pelvic hole. Normally, the pelvi organs are held in place by these muscles and related tissues The rectum, uterus, and bladder are some of these organs However, age, childbirth, pregnancy, and specific surgica procedures might weaken these muscles.

All women need to understand the significance of the pelvi floor. In addition to preventing incontinence, a strong pelvi floor is necessary for sexual health, core stability, and genera well-being.

This book is structured with multiple sections, eacl addressing a distinct facet of pelvic floor health. The commor issues that might result from having a weak pelvic floor wil be discussed after providing an outline of the anatomy anc function of the pelvic floor.

Next, we'll explore the many kinds of pelvic floor exercises or Kegel exercises that work to strengthen these muscles anc reduce symptoms.

his book is for any woman, whether she is a young lady interested in preventive healthcare, a new mother recuperating from childbirth, or a woman exhibiting symptoms associated with a weak pelvic floor.

Our goal is to empower you to take charge of your pelvic health and gain a greater understanding of your body by offering accurate, succinct, and understandable information.

Never forget that strengthening your pelvic floor can begin at any time. So let's set off on this path to greater health and a higher standard of living together. Welcome aboard!

Pelvic Floor Exercises

Exercises for strengthening the pelvic floor muscles are referred to as pelvic floor exercises, or Kegel exercises.

The pelvic organs, which include the urethra, rectum, bladder, intestines, and, in females, the vagina, cervix, and uterus, are supported by these muscles.

How to Perform Pelvic Floor Exercises

Consult a healthcare professional before beginning pelvic floor exercises to make sure your symptoms are caused by weak or tight muscles rather than an underlying medical condition. The following workout can be beneficial:

1. Diaphragmatic Breathing, Or Deep Breathing:

This practice eases tension in the pelvic floor and other muscles throughout the body. Additionally, it lessens the discomfort that tight pelvic floor muscles may produce.

1. On a solid surface, lie on your back.

2. Put your feet level on the ground and bend your knees.

3. Put a hand on your belly and another on your chest.

4. Inhale slowly through your nose, allowing the oxygen to fill your belly. The hand on your chest should

remain motionless, while the hand on your stomach should rise.

5. Blow out the air gently by shaping your lips to resemble a candle being blown out.

6. Do this for five breaths.

oles of Pelvic Floor Exercises on the Woman's ody

xercises targeting the pelvic floor are very important for a oman's body.

Preventing Incontinence: Both fecal and urine continence can be avoided with a strong pelvic floor.

Sexual Health: Both sexes can benefit from these activities terms of improved sexual function.

Core Stability: The muscles that make up the core group, hich includes the pelvic floor muscles, give the body ability.

Pregnancy and Childbirth: A strong pelvic floor can ipport a woman both throughout labor and her postpartum cuperation.

Preventing Pelvic Organ Prolapse: By making these uscles stronger, you can stop pelvic organ prolapse, a

condition in which the organs in your pelvis fall out of yo
body as a result of weak muscles.

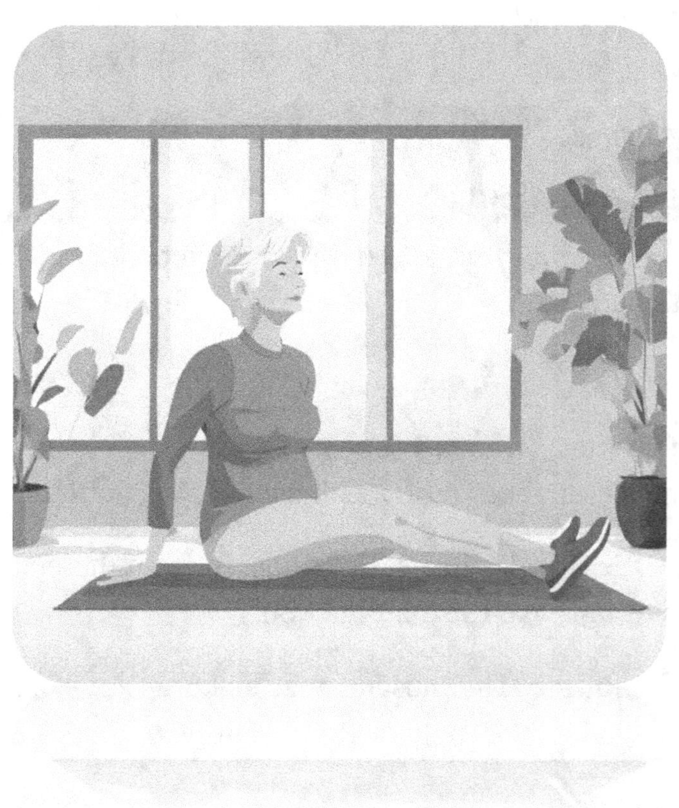

Understanding the Anatomy of the Pelvic Floor

Understanding the anatomy of the pelvic floor is essential for anyone seeking to optimize their pelvic health and well-being. The pelvic floor is a complex network of muscles, ligaments, and connective tissues that form the base of the pelvis. It serves several crucial functions, including supporting the pelvic organs, maintaining urinary and fecal continence, stabilizing the pelvis, and contributing to sexual function.

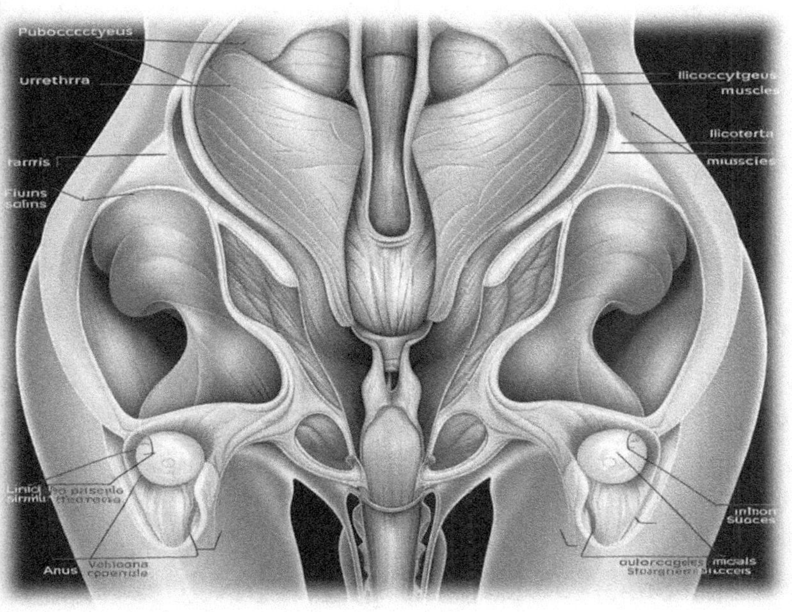

To ascertain the pelvic floor's anatomy comprehensively, let'
break it down into its constituent components:

1. Muscles:

The pelvic floor muscles are made up of multiple layers, eac
with specific attachments and roles. There are two layers t
these muscles: superficial and deep.

Muscles like the bulbospongiosus, ischiocavernosus, an
superficial transverse perineal muscles are found in th
superficial layer. These muscles are involved in the suppor
and function of sexuality.

Muscles like the puborectalis, iliococcygeus, an
pubococcygeus are found in the deep layer. These muscle
maintain the pelvic organs structurally and aid in fecal an
urine continence.

2. Ligaments and Connective Tissues:

These anatomical structures offer the pelvic organs stability
and support. The uterosacral ligaments, pubocervical fascia
and sacrotuberous ligaments are some of the structures tha
aid in holding the uterus, vagina, and bladder in place.

Additionally, these tissues are essential for preserving
pelvic organ prolapse and avoiding incontinence.

. Pelvic Organs:

he bladder, uterus, vagina, and rectum are just a few of the
ssential organs for which the pelvic floor acts as a
undamental support system.

Maintaining these organs in the ideal posture and
unctioning requires the pelvic floor to operate properly.
rinary incontinence, pelvic organ prolapse, and pelvic pain
yndromes are just a few of the pelvic floor disorders that can
sult from dysfunction in the pelvic floor muscles or
upporting structures.

. Nerve Supply:

complex network of nerves, including branches of the
acral plexus and pudendal nerve, make up the pelvic floor.

These neurons give the pelvic floor muscles sensory and
motor abilities, enabling voluntary control over sexual feeling
nd fecal and urine continence.

. Blood flow:

he tissues and muscles of the pelvic floor depend on a
ufficient blood flow to remain healthy.

The internal iliac artery branches supply blood to the pelv
floor muscles and organs, facilitating healthy nutrient an
oxygenation.

The basis for efficient pelvic floor rehabilitation, exercis
routine, and management of pelvic floor problems is a
understanding of the anatomy of the pelvic floor.

It makes it possible for people to become more cognizant c
their bodies, spot possible problems, and take preventativ
action to enhance pelvic health and general wellbeing.

Importance of Pelvic Floor Health for Women

ecause the pelvic floor supports many vital physiological
unctions, it is imperative to maintain its health.

Vital Functions of the Pelvic Floor

. Supports Pelvic Organs:

he bladder, uterus, prostate, and rectum are among the
elvic organs that the pelvic floor muscles support. These
rgans need this support in order to function properly.

. Stabilizes the Pelvis and Spine:

o support the pelvis and spine, the pelvic floor muscles
ollaborate with the deep abdominal and deep back muscles.

. Supports Sexual Function:

oth sexual function and satisfaction are influenced by a
ealthy pelvic floor.

4. Supports Bladder and Bowel Control:

The muscles of the pelvic floor are essential for bladder and bowel control. Having weak muscles can result incontinence.

The Importance of Healthy Pelvic Floor

1. Prevention of Pelvic Floor Disorders:

Incontinence, pelvic pain, pelvic pressure, sexual dysfunction and prolapse of the pelvic organs affect up to 25% of adult population. Frequent pelvic floor exercises can aid in the avoidance of these conditions.

2. Readying for Childbirth and Recovery:

Having a strong pelvic floor helps support you both throughout labor and after giving birth.

3. Sexual Health:

Enhancing sexual performance and happiness is possible with a healthy pelvic floor.

4. Incontinence Prevention:

Frequent pelvic floor exercises will stop both fecal and urinary incontinence.

General Well-Being:

General well-being and life quality are enhanced by a healthy pelvic floor.

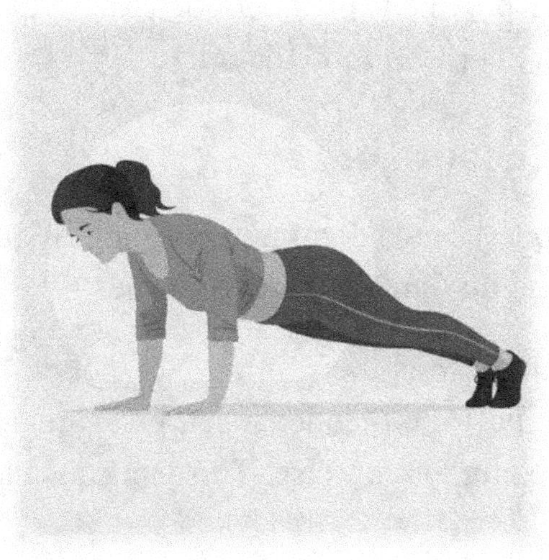

Pelvic Floor Problems

Recognizing the symptoms, getting the right therapy, and enhancing overall pelvic health all depend on your ability to understand the prevalent pelvic floor issues. Let's examine a few of these concerns in more detail:

1. Urinary Incontinence:

This pelvic floor issue is common, particularly in women, and is defined as the involuntary flow of urine.

Stress incontinence is the result of the pelvic floor muscles inability to support the bladder when pressure builds up from coughing, sneezing, or exercise. This can cause leakage.

Urge incontinence, sometimes referred to as overactive bladder, is characterized by an intense, unexpected urge to urinate that frequently leads to leaks before going to the bathroom.

Mixed Incontinences is when stress and urge incontinence symptoms are combined

2. Pelvic Organ Prolapse:

Pelvic organ prolapse is the condition in which the bladder, uterus, or rectum bulge into the vagina after falling from their natural position.

Pelvic organ prolapse can be caused by aging, obesity, connective tissue weakness, childbearing, and other factors.

A feeling of fullness or pressure in the pelvic region, tissue extending from the vagina, fecal or urine incontinence, and discomfort during sexual activity are some of the possible symptoms.

Pelvic Pain Syndromes:

These conditions include endometriosis, vulvodynia, interstitial cystitis/bladder pain syndrome (IC/BPS), and chronic pelvic pain syndrome (CPPS), among other chronic pain illnesses involving the pelvic region.

These disorders can result in lower back, pelvic, vaginal, or lower abdomen pain that is chronic and frequently incapacitating. Other symptoms that may accompany these ailments include urgency or frequent urination as well as discomfort during sexual activity.

Dyspareunia (Painful Intercourse):

Dyspareunia is the term for ongoing pain during sexual activity. It can be caused by a number of things, such as hormone imbalances, dry vagina, pelvic floor muscle dysfunction, or underlying medical issues.

Dyspareunia can be caused by weak or tight pelvic floor muscles, which can lead to muscle spasms or insufficient support for the pelvic organs.

5. Constipation and Defecation difficulties:

The inability of the pelvic floor muscles to coordinate an
relax during bowel motions is known as pelvic floc
dysfunction. This condition can lead to chronic constipatic
and defecation difficulties.

A sensation of obstruction or blockage in the rectur
straining during bowel motions, difficulty passing stools, ar
partial evacuation are some of the symptoms that may t
experienced.

6. Sexual Dysfunction:

Issues with arousal, orgasm, or pain during sexual activity a
some of the ways that pelvic floor dysfunction can present a
sexual dysfunction.

Sexual dysfunction in women can be caused by a variety c
conditions, including nerve injury, hormone imbalance
pelvic floor muscle tightness, and psychological issues.

Starting Pelvic Floor Exercises

for Women

ee a doctor before beginning pelvic floor exercises to make
ure your symptoms are caused by tightness or weakness in
our muscles rather than an underlying medical condition like
adder issues or pelvic organ prolapse, which is the dropping
f the pelvic organs due to muscle weakness.

ot everyone is a good candidate for Kegel exercises, or
elvic floor exercises. Kegel exercises can help strengthen the
elvic floor, but they can exacerbate tight muscles.

reparing for effective pelvic floor exercises involves several
ey steps to ensure safety, comfort, and optimal results.

ollowing clearance, take into account the following
reparations:

. Educate Yourself:

vest some time in learning about the structure and purposes
f the pelvic floor muscles. Your awareness during exercises
ill be improved if you are aware of the anatomy of the

pelvic floor and how it functions in relation to the bladder, bowel, and sexual system.

2. Pelvic Floor Assessment:

You might want to think about getting a pelvic floor assessment from a pelvic floor physical therapist or women's health specialist. This evaluation can assist in locating any muscular dysfunction, tension, or weakness that would require special attention when performing workouts.

3. Proper Breathing Techniques:

As diaphragmatic breathing is essential for pelvic floor exercises, learn and practice it. It is possible to improve both muscular engagement and relaxation by synchronizing your breath with pelvic floor contractions.

4. Maintain Nutrition and Hydration:

To support overall pelvic health, eat a balanced diet high in fiber and drink enough of water. Consuming a healthy diet and being hydrated can help avoid constipation, which can worsen pelvic floor issues.

5. Comfortable Clothes:

To promote correct muscle engagement and range of motion during pelvic floor exercises, wear loose, comfortable clothing.

6. Establish a Calm Environment:

Look for a peaceful, well-lit area where you may concentrate on your pelvic floor exercises without being interrupted. Setting up a peaceful space might help you practice mindfulness and relaxation.

7. Pelvic Floor Awareness:

To connect with and comprehend the feeling of activating and relaxing your pelvic floor muscles, practice pelvic floor awareness exercises. Enhancing consciousness of pelvic floor sensations can be achieved through the use of mindfulness practices including body scanning and visualization.

8. Start Slowly and Advance Gradually:

As your strength and control improve, start with mild pelvic floor exercises like Kegels and progressively increase the complexity, length, and intensity. Stay away from overdoing it and pay attention to your body.

9. Consistency and Persistence:

Make pelvic floor exercises a regular part of your practice by putting them into your daily schedule. To improve and preserve the health of the pelvic floor over time, consistency is essential.

10. Track Progress and Adjustments:

Document any changes in pelvic floor function or symptoms
as well as your progress. As your body and your healthcare
provider provide feedback, modify your workout routine as
necessary.

Pilate Exercises for Pelvic Floor Health

. Pelvic Tilts:

1. Lay flat on your back with your feet flat and your knees bent.
2. Breathe in to get ready, and then release the breath as you raise your pelvis and contract your pelvic floor muscles.
3. Inhale to return to neutral.
4. Repeat over ten times.

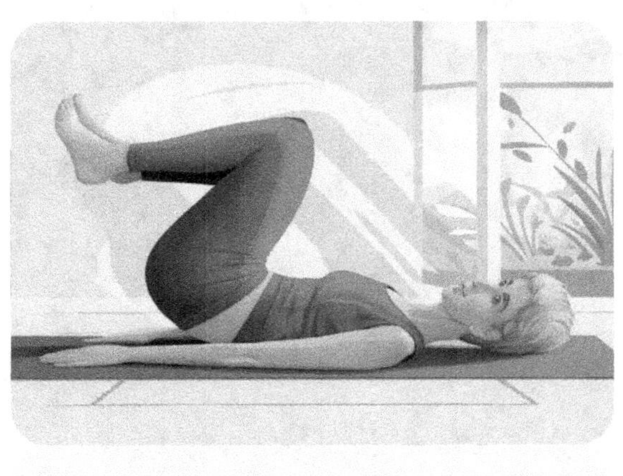

2. Bridge with Squeeze:

1. Start in the pelvic tilting posture.

2. Squeeze your pelvic floor muscles while lifting your
    hips into a bridge position.

3. Reposition and repeat ten times.

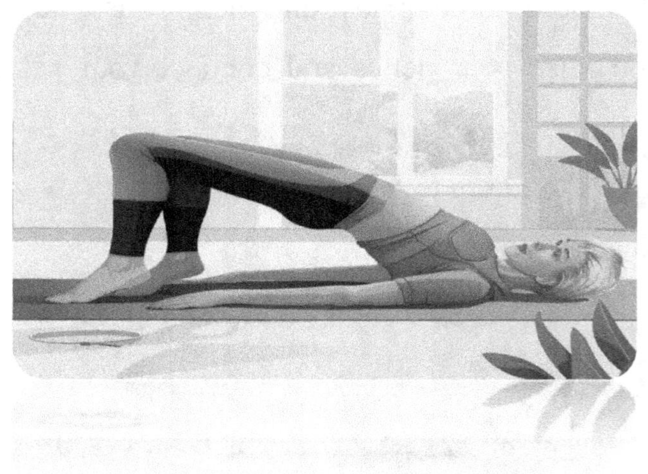

Supine Kegels:

1. Lie on your back with your feet flat and knees bent down or up.
2. Take a deep breath, release it, and contract your pelvic floor muscles as though you're halting the flow of pee.
3. Release after five seconds of holding.
4. Repeat over ten times.

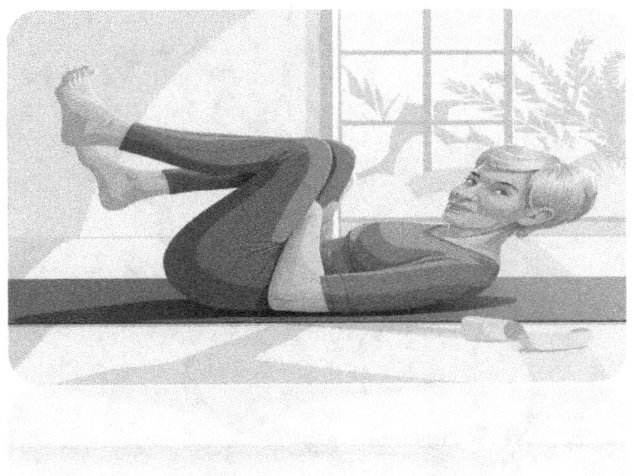

4. Standing Pelvic Clock:

1. Stand with your feet hip-width apart.

2. Picture a clock underneath your feet.

3. Tilt your pelvis forward starting at 12 o'clock, the work your way around the clock to 3 o'clock, o'clock, and 9 o'clock.

4. Five clockwise and five counterclockwise repetition are to be done.

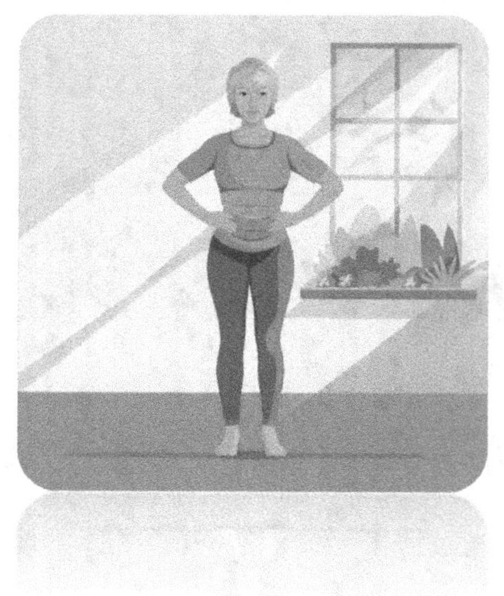

. Pelvic Floor Activators:

1. Sit tall on a chair or stability ball.

2. Breathe in deeply, and then release the air while you gently elevate and tense your pelvic floor muscles without using your abdominals or glutes.

3. Five seconds of holding, then release.

4. Repeat over ten times.

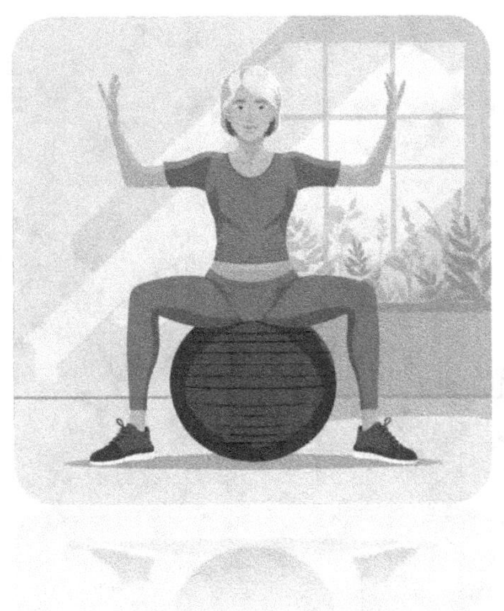

6. Pelvic Floor Lifts:

1. Lie on your back with your knees bent and feet flat o
    legs up.

2. Breathe in to prepare, and then exhale as you attemp
    to draw your pelvic floor muscles up toward you
    head.

3. Five seconds of holding, then release.

4. Repeat over ten times.

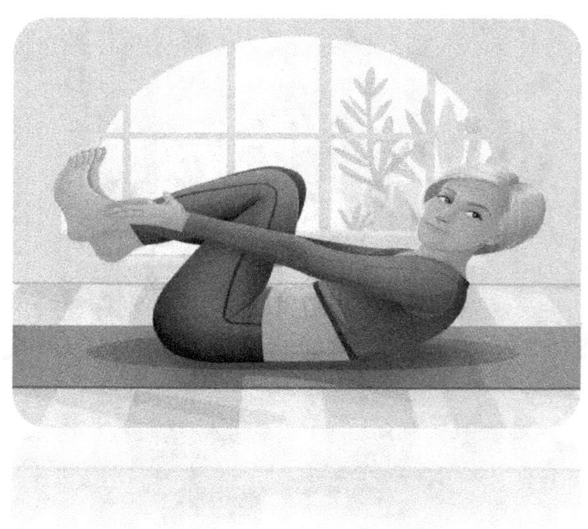

. Pelvic Floor Walks:

1. Take a seat and place your feet flat on the ground.

2. Think of the floor of your pelvis like an elevator.

3. Breathe in to warm up, and then exhale as you raise your pelvic floor muscles gradually, like you're walking up floors.

4. Release each level separately.

5. Repeat over five times.

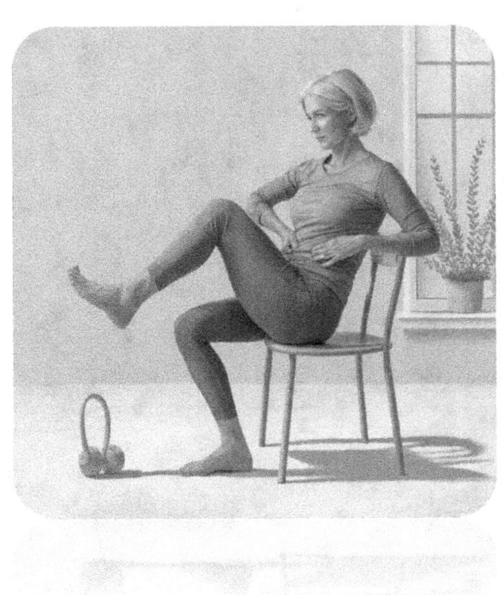

8. Pelvic Floor Coordination:

1. Place your feet hip-width apart and stand tall.

2. Take a deep breath, release it as you lift one leg forward and contract your pelvic floor muscles.

3. Repeat with the other leg after lowering the first.

4. Repeat ten times with different legs.

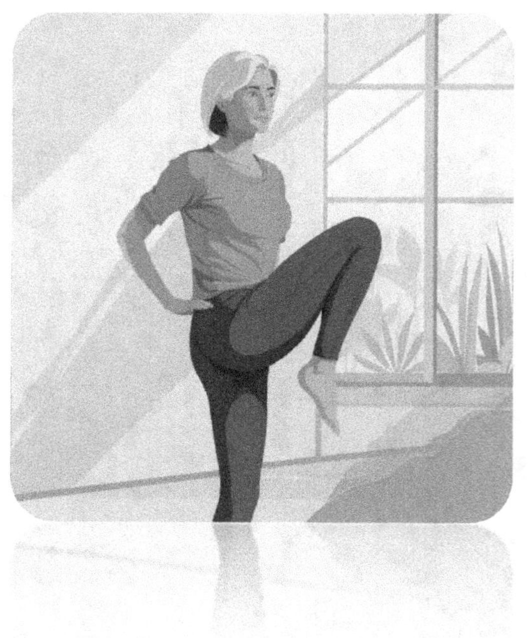

. Heel Slides with Pelvic Floor Engagement:

1. Lay flat on your back with your feet flat and your knees bent.

2. Breathe in to prepare, and then exhale as your pelvic floor muscles contract.

3. Slowly move one heel along the floor and once the leg is straight then return to the beginning position.

4. Alternate legs for 10 repetitions per leg.

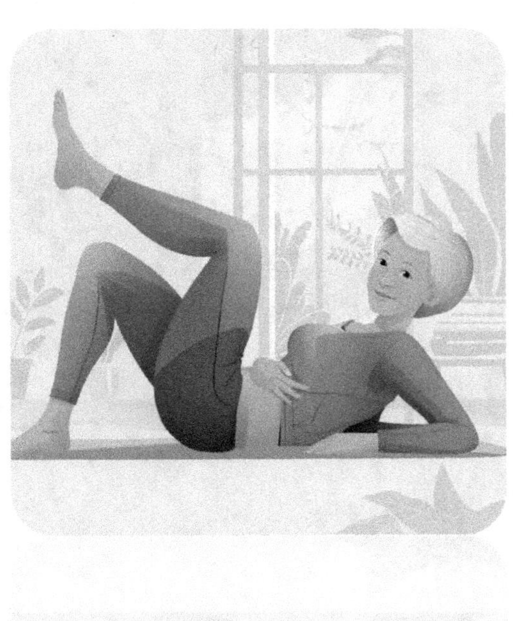

10. Tabletop with Pelvic Floor Activation:

1. Lay flat on your back, shins parallel to the floor and knees bent.

2. Breathe in to prepare, and then exhale as you lift one foot off the ground and draw the knee in toward your chest by using your pelvic floor muscles.

3. Do ten repetitions of each leg switching positions.

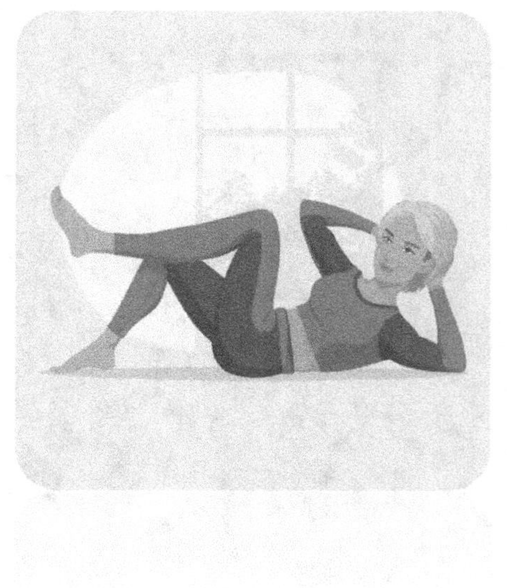

1. Pelvic Floor Squats:

1. Place your feet slightly wider than hip-width apart.

2. Breathe in deeply, and then release the breath as you lower yourself into a squat by using your pelvic floor muscles.

3. Take a breath to stand back up.

4. Repeat over ten times.

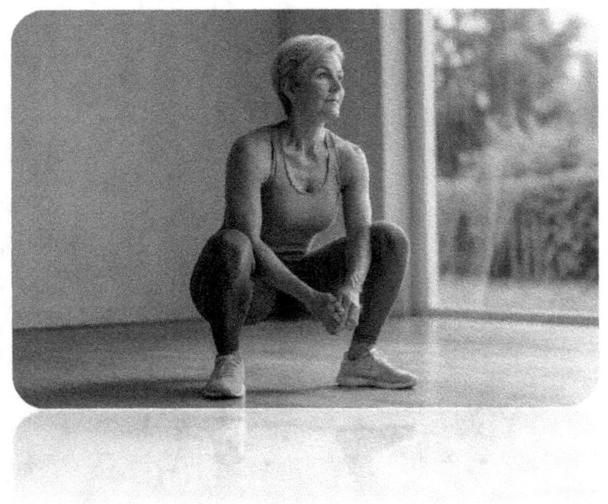

12. Pelvic Floor Step-Ups:

1. Take a stance in front of a sturdy platform or set o
   steps.

2. Breathe in deeply, and then release the breath as you
   step one foot onto the platform and contract you
   pelvic floor muscles.

3. Retrace your steps and use the opposite foot.

4. Do ten repetitions of each leg switching positions.

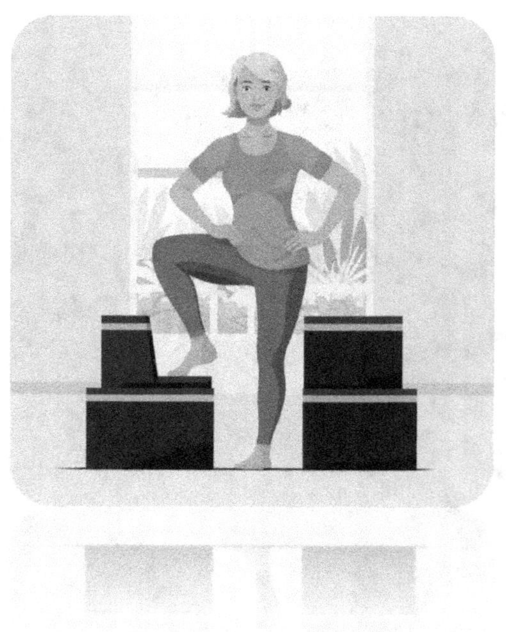

Pelvic Floor Side Leg Lifts:

1. Lie on your side, legs extended and stacked on top of one another.

2. Breathe in to get ready, and then exhale as you raise your upper leg toward the ceiling by using your pelvic floor muscles.

3. Repeat ten times on each side after lowering the leg.

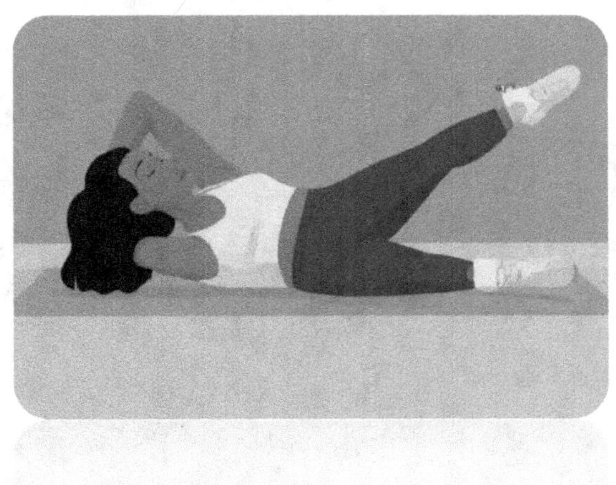

14. Pelvic Floor Plank:

1. Begin in a plank position, with your body erect from head to heels and your hands directly beneath your shoulders.

2. Take a deep breath; release it while you contract your pelvic floor muscles.

3. Hold for ten to twenty seconds, then let go.

4. Do this three times.

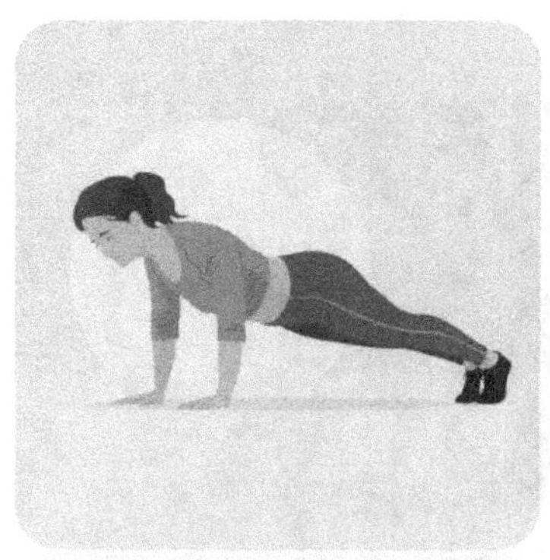 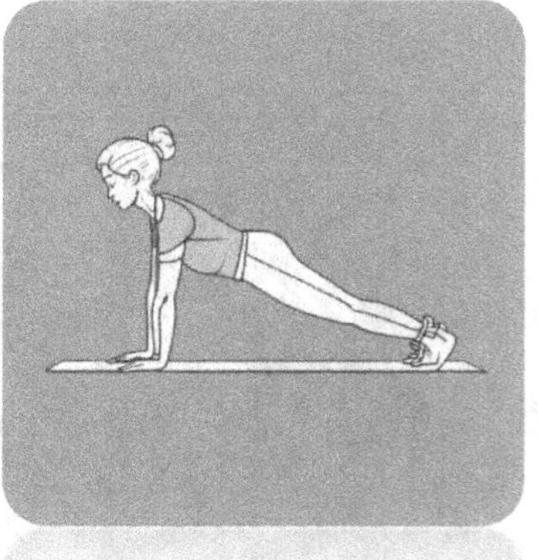

5. Pelvic Floor Roll-Ups:

1. Lay flat on your back, arms raised above your head, and legs outstretched.

2. Breathe in to warm up, then release as you contract your pelvic floor muscles and raise your spine one vertebra at a time to a seated position.

3. To get back to where you were before, reverse the motion.

4. Repeat over ten times.

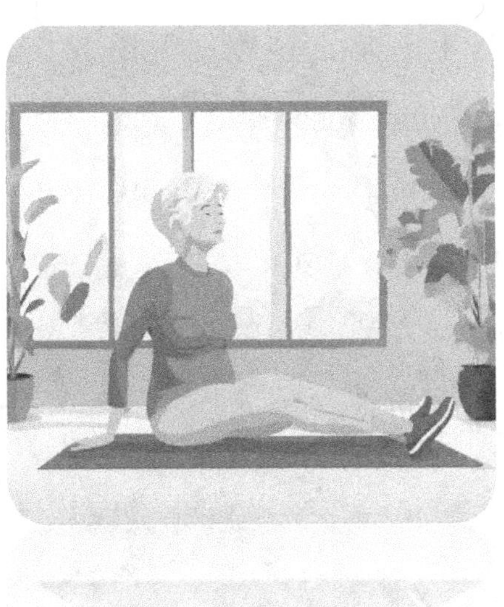

Core Exercises for Pelvic Floor Health

1. Pelvic Tilt Plank:

1. Begin in a plank position, with your body in a straight line from head to heels and your hands directly beneath your shoulders.

2. Pull your belly button in the direction of your spine and gently lift your pelvic floor to engage your core and pelvic floor muscles.

3. While keeping your breathing constant, hold this position for 30 to 1 minute.

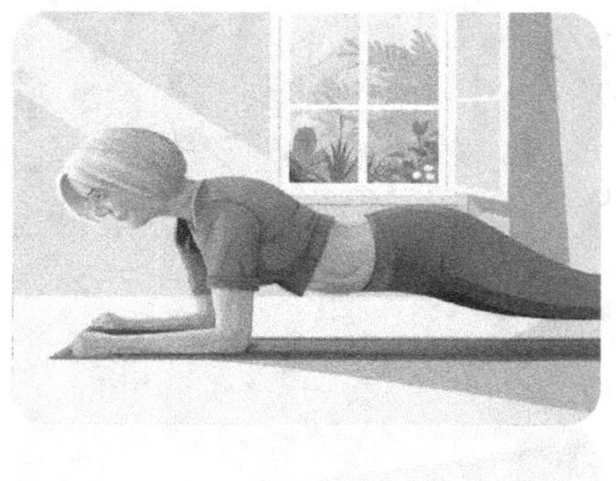

2. Dead Bug:

1. Assume a lying position, extending your arms skyward and positioning your legs like a tabletop (knees bent at a 90-degree angle).
2. When you descend one arm and the other leg toward the floor, contract your pelvic floor and core muscles.
3. Go back to the beginning and repeat on the opposite side.
4. For ten to twelve repetitions on each side, switch sides.

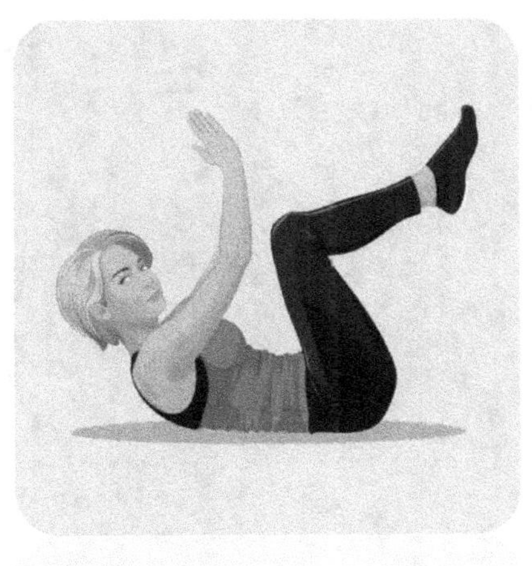

3. Bird Dog (Arms Only):

1. Place your wrists under your shoulders and your knee under your hips to begin this tabletop pose.

2. Maintaining your hips and shoulders level, stretch one arm straight out in front of you and one leg stretched out behind you, parallel to the floor, while contracting your core muscles.

3. Hold for a little while before switching sides and going back to the beginning position.

4. Do ten to twelve repetitions on each side while concentrating on control and stability.

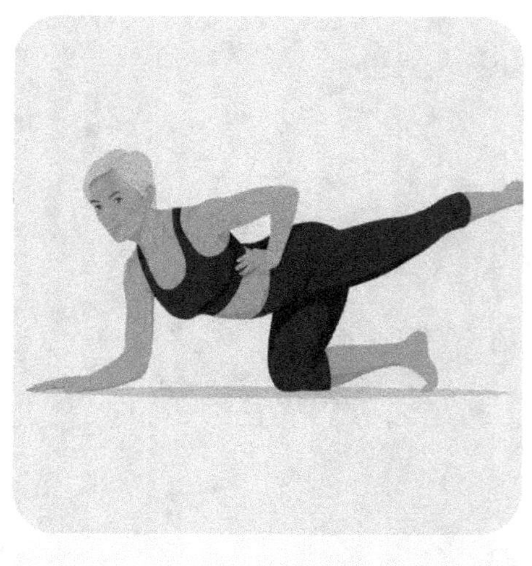

Side Plank:

1. Lie on your side with your legs stacked on top of one another and your elbow directly beneath your shoulder.

2. Lift your hips off the ground and make a straight line from your head to your heels by using your pelvic floor and core muscles.

3. Maintain this posture for 30 to 60 seconds on each side.

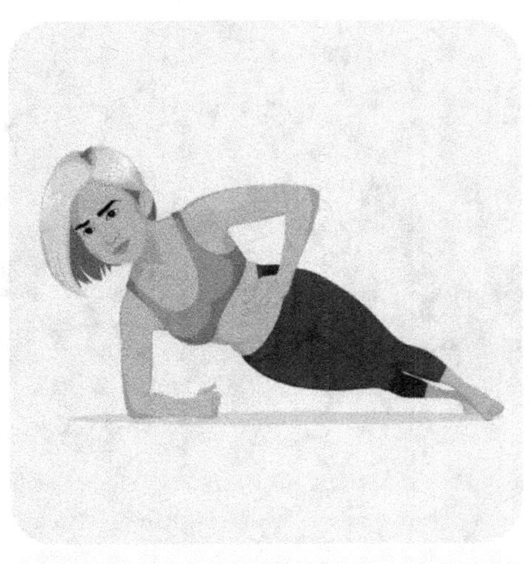

5. Modified Leg Raises:

1. While lying on your back, extend your legs straigh
   and place your hands by your sides.
2. Maintaining your legs straight as you raise both towar
   the ceiling, contract your pelvic floor and co
   muscles.
3. Without allowing your raised legs make contact wit
   the floor, slowly lower your legs back down toward
   the floor.
4. Do 10–12 repeats of this.

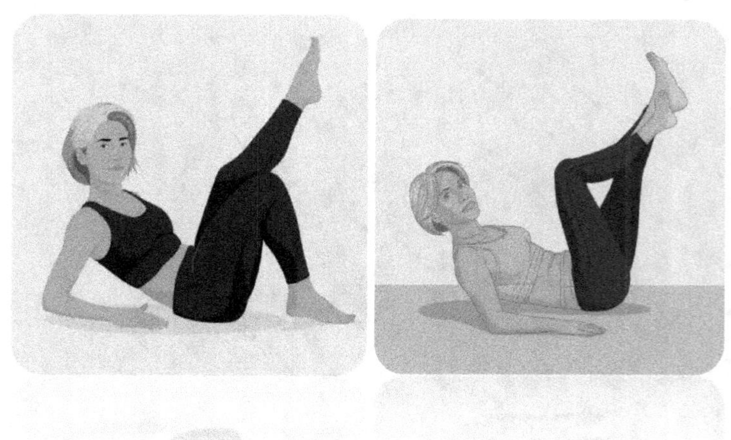

1. Hold a weight or medicine ball in front of your chest while sitting on the floor with your knees bent and your feet flat on the floor.
2. Lift your feet off the ground and lean back slightly while using your pelvic floor and core muscles.
3. Turn your body to the right and shift your weight to the floor in front of your right hip.
4. After circling back to the middle, turn to the left.
5. Do ten to twelve repetitions on each side.

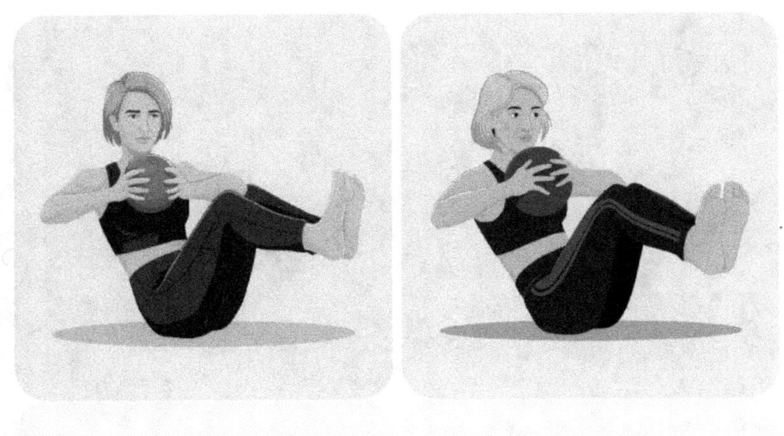

7. Mountain Climbers:

1. Begin in a plank position, with your body erect from head to heels and your hands directly beneath your shoulders.
2. As you drive one knee toward your chest, contract your pelvic floor and core muscles.
3. Then, rapidly switch legs to begin sprinting.
4. Keep switching legs quickly for duration of 30 to 6 seconds.

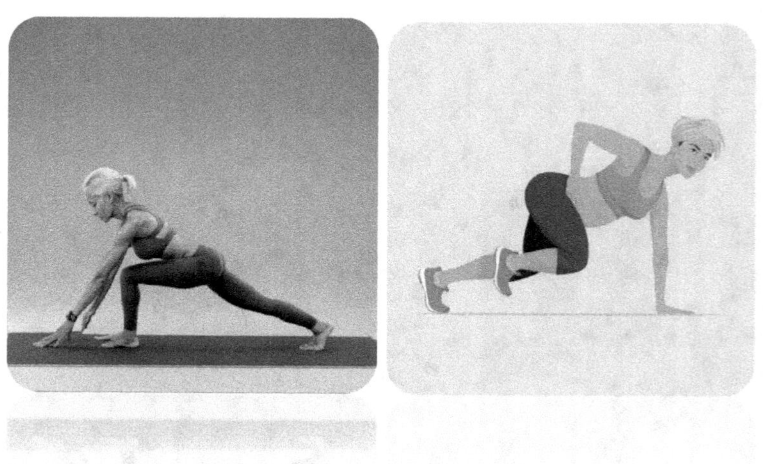

8. Side Plank with Hip Dip:

1. Begin in a forearm plank position, with your elbows exactly beneath your shoulders and your body in a straight.

2. As you twist your hips to the right and dipping them towards the floor, contract your pelvic floor and core muscles.

3. Take a step back to the middle and turn your hips to the left.

4. Do ten to twelve repetitions on each side.

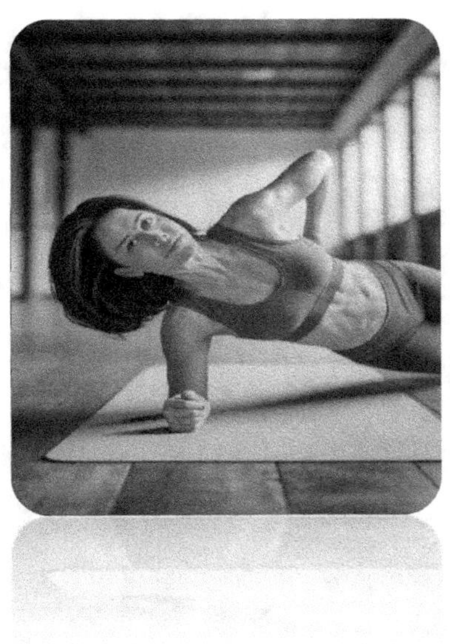

9. Bicycle Crunches:

1. Place your legs up in a tabletop posture while lying on your back with your hands behind your head.

2. As you pull your right elbow toward your left knee while simultaneously straightening your right leg, contract your pelvic floor and core muscles.

3. Continue in a pedaling motion, alternating on the opposite side.

4. Do 10–12 repetitions on each side.

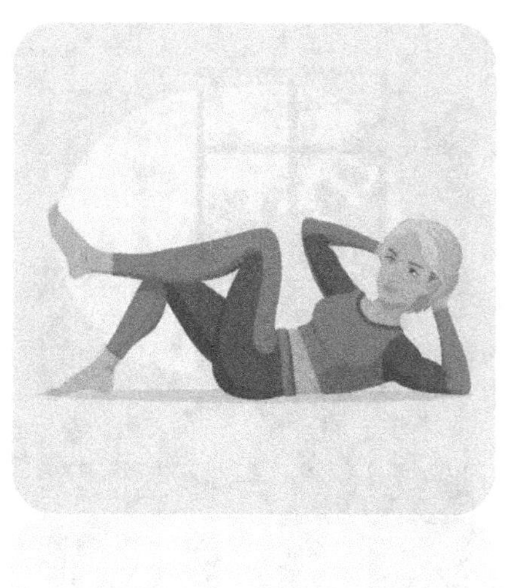

0. Plank with Knee-to-Elbow:

1. Begin in a plank posture, keeping your body in a straight line and your hands directly beneath your shoulders.
2. Squeeze your obliques while bringing your right knee up to your right elbow by using your core and pelvic floor muscles.
3. Go back to the beginning and repeat on the opposite side.
4. For ten to twelve repetitions on each side, switch sides.

1. Pilates Hundred:

1. Lie on your back with your arms at your sides, knees bent, and feet flat on the ground.
2. As you raise your head, shoulders, and neck off the mat and extend your arms toward your feet, contract your pelvic floor and core muscles.
3. Breathe in for five counts, out for five counts, and pump your arms up and down in a controlled motion to complete 100 arm pumps.

12. Boat Pose:

1. Sit on the floor with your hands lying next to your hips, your knees bent, and your feet flat on the floor.

2. As you elevate your feet off the ground and lean back slightly to balance on your sit bones, contract your pelvic floor and core muscles.

3. Stretch your arms straight ahead of you, keeping them parallel to the ground.

4. Maintain this posture for duration of 30 to 1 minute.

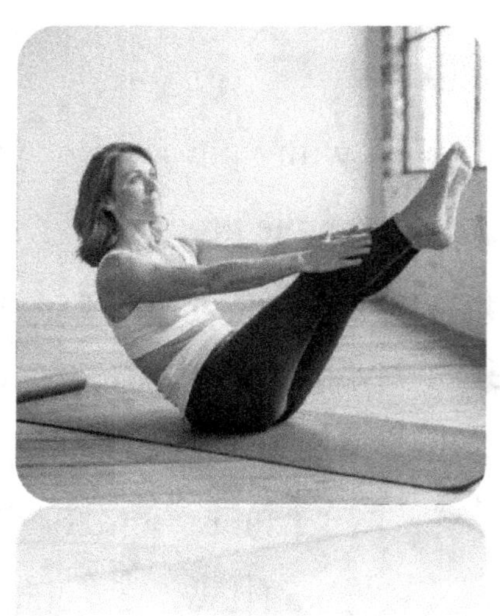

3. Modified Side Plank:

1. Place your elbow just behind your shoulder while lying on your side with your knees bent.

2. Lift your hips off the ground and make a straight line from your head to your knees by using your pelvic floor and core muscles.

3. Maintain this posture for 30 to 60 seconds on each side.

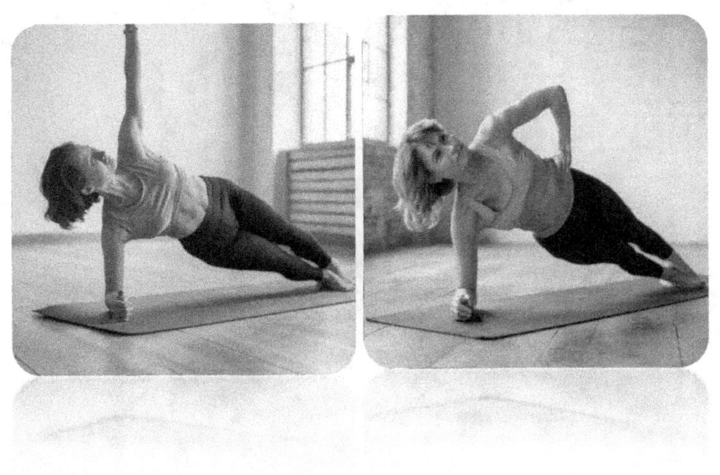

14. Reverse Crunches:

1. Lie on your back with your arms by your sides, knee bent, and feet flat on the ground.
2. As you raise your knees toward your chest and rais your hips off the ground, contract your pelvic floor an core muscles.
3. Control fully lower your legs back down to the floor.
4. Do 10–12 repeats of this.

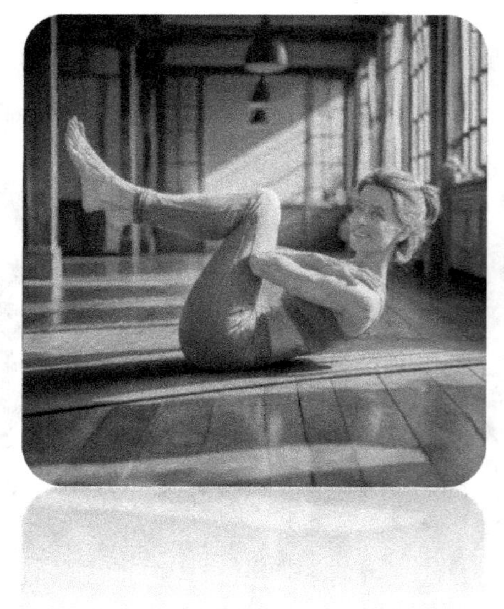

15. Superman Pose:

1. Place your arms high and your legs straight while lying face down on the mat.

2. As you simultaneously raise your arms, chest, and legs off the ground, contract your pelvic floor and core muscles.

3. After a little period of holding this position, lower back down.

4. Do 10–12 repeats of this.

Yoga Poses for Pelvic Floor Health

1. Bound Angle Pose (Baddha Konasana):

1. Sit on the floor with your knees out to the sides. Bring the soles of your feet together.
2. Sit up straight, stretching your spine, and hold your feet with your hands.
3. Breathe deeply and use your pelvic floor muscles to hold the pose for 30s to 1 minute.

2. Warrior II Pose (Virabhadrasana II):

1. Place your feet wide apart, pointing one foot forward and inwardly pointing the other.
2. While maintaining a firm, straight back leg, bend your front knee to a 90-degree angle.
3. Extend your arms sideways, keeping them parallel to the ground, and look over your front digits.

4. Hold this position for 30 to 60 seconds while using your pelvic floor muscles.

5. Continue on the opposite side.

. Chair Pose (Utkatasana):

1. Stand with your arms at your sides and your feet together.

2. Taking a breath, raise your arms upward with your palms facing one another.

3. Breathe out as you lower your hips and bend your knees, as if sitting back into a chair.

4. Contract your pelvic floor muscles, and then hold them for duration of 30s to 60 seconds.

4. Cat-Cow Stretch:

1. Begin on your hands and knees, placing your knees beneath your hips and your wrists directly beneath your shoulders.

2. Take a breath and raise your tailbone and chest toward the ceiling while arching your back (Cow Pose).

3. Release your breath as you circle your spine, bringing your tailbone down, and burying your chin into your chest (cat pose).

4. Continue for five to ten cycles, synchronizing your movements with your breathing.

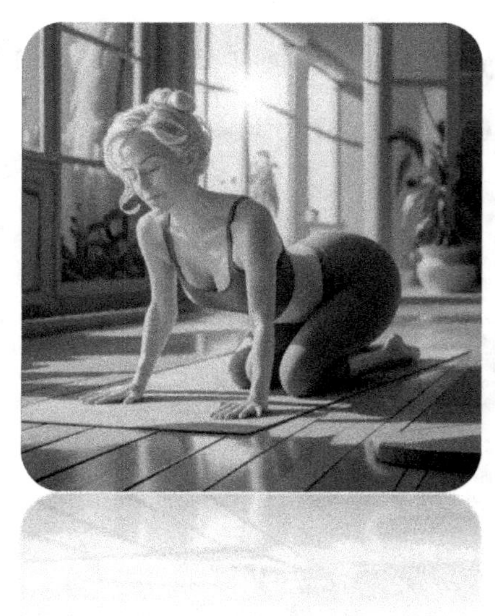

. Low Lunge (Anjaneyasana):

1. This is done from a standing position.

2. Step backward with one foot into a lunge, keeping the back knee on the floor.

3. Sink your hips toward the floor while maintaining your front knee stacked over your ankle.

4. Lift your chest and contract your pelvic floor muscles.

5. Hold for 30s to 1 minute.

6. Continue on the opposite side.

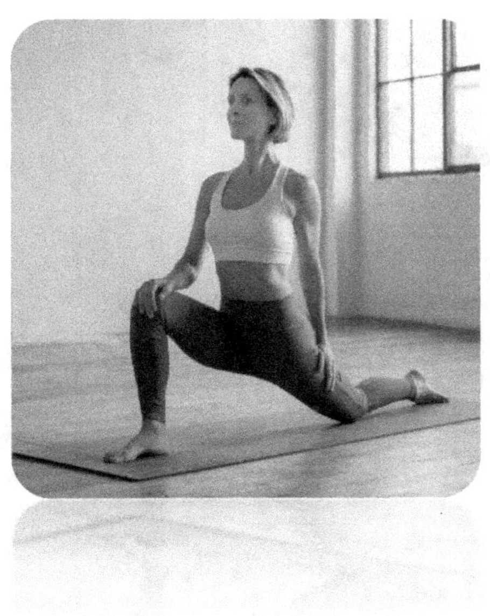

6.   Upward-Facing   Dog   (Urdhva   Mukh Svanasana):

1. Begin by lying face down on the mat with your elbow bent and your palms by your sides.
2. Take a breath, press into your hands, raise your thigh and chest off the mat, and straighten your arms.
3. Engage your pelvic floor muscles while lowering an keeping your shoulders away from your ears.
4. Hold for 30s to 1 minute.

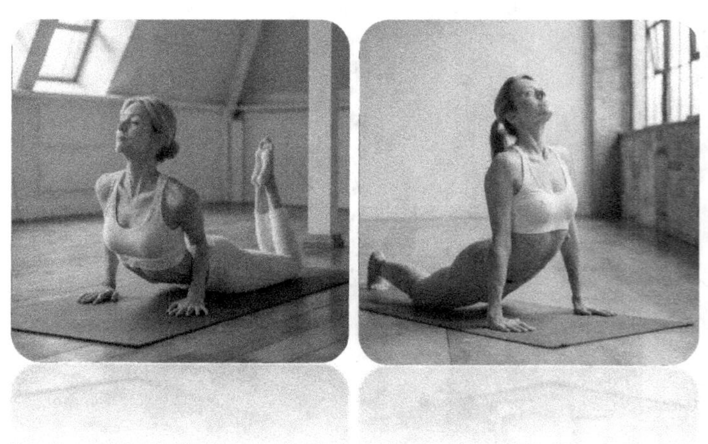

. Child's Pose (Balasana):

1. Begin on your hands and knees, and then sit back on your heels with your knees apart.

2. Extend your arms in front of you or place them by your sides as you fold inward and lower your chest toward the floor.

3. Breathe deeply and with relaxation, noticing a slight stretch in your hips and using your pelvic floor muscles.

4. Hold for one to three minutes.

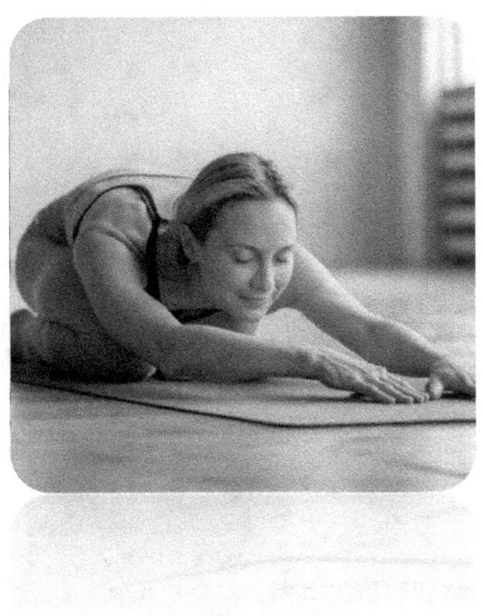

8. Tree Pose (Vrksasana):

1. Exhale fully, place your arms by your sides, and stand tall with your feet hip-width apart.

2. Transfer your weight on one foot, lift the other, and press the sole of the elevated foot against the inside of your standing leg's thigh or calf.

3. To activate your pelvic floor muscles, press your foot into your thigh or calf and your thigh or calf into your foot.

4. Hold for 30s to 1 minute.

5. Continue on the opposite side.

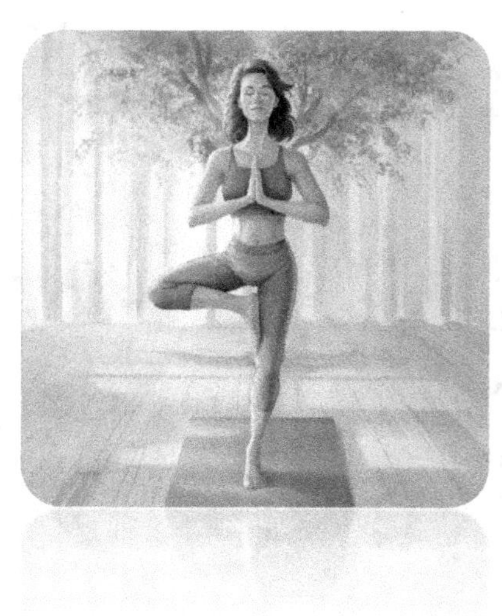

. King Cobra Pose (Bhujangasana):

1. Place your palms by your sides and bend your elbows while lying face down on the mat.
2. Breathe in as you press into your palms and raise your chest off the mat while maintaining a grounded pelvis.
3. Engage your pelvic floor muscles while lowering and keeping your shoulders away from your ears.
4. Hold for 30s to 1 minute.

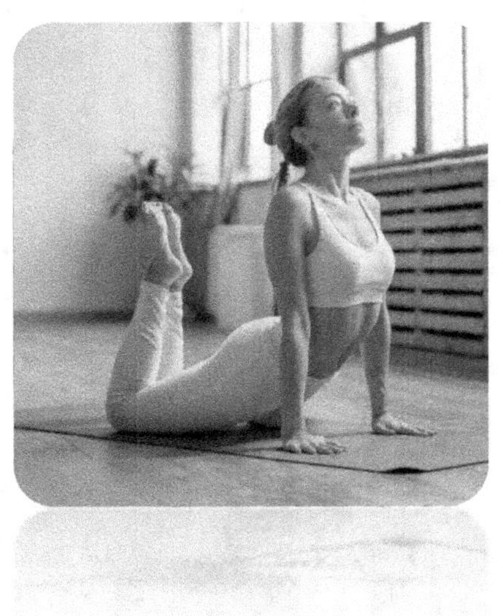

10. Downward-Facing Dog (Adho Mukh Svanasana):

1. Begin on your hands and knees, placing your knee behind your hips and your wrists directly beneath you shoulders.
2. Form an inverted V shape with your body by tuckin your toes, lifting your hips toward the ceiling, an straightening your legs.
3. As you lengthen through your spine, firmly press you hands into the mat and contract your pelvic floc muscles.
4. Hold for 30s to 1 minute.

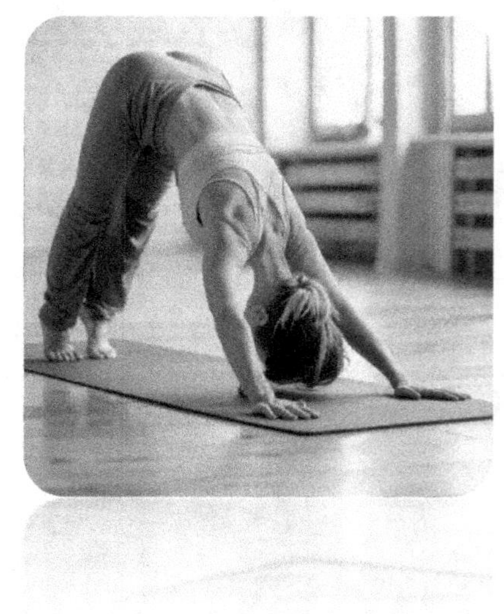

1. Pigeon Pose (Eka Pada Rajakapotasana):

1. Begin in plank position.
2. Then, bring your right knee to your right wrist and place your right ankle next to your left wrist.
3. Keep your spine long and contract your pelvic floor muscles as you slide your left leg back, straightening the knee and lowering your hips toward the mat.
4. Repeat on the opposite side after holding for 30s to 1 minute.

2. Supine Twist (Supta Matsyendrasana):

1. Assume a lying position on your back and extend your arms in a T-shape out to the sides.
2. Bring your knees up to your chest by bending them.
3. While maintaining your shoulders firmly planted, lower both of your knees to the right side of your body.
4. Look over your left shoulder and contract your pelvic floor muscles.
5. Repeat on the opposite side after holding for 30s to 1 minute.

Other Necessary Exercises

1. Deep Breathing (Diaphragmatic Breathing):

1. Place your feet firmly on the floor and bend you
   knees while lying on your back.

2. Grasp your abdomen with one hand and your che
   with the other.

3. Breathe in deeply through your nostrils, allowing you
   abdomen to expand as the air fills your lungs.

4. Breathe out slowly through your lips, letting your bell
   drop as your lungs are cleared.

5. As you breathe, concentrate on letting your pelvi
   floor muscles relax.

2. Quick Flick Kegels:

1. With your feet flat on the floor and your knees bent, li
   down.

2. Squeeze and raise your pelvic floor muscles rapidly, a
   though you're halting the flow of pee.

3. After holding the contraction for one to two seconds, let go and fully relax.

4. Ten to fifteen times, repeat this brief contraction-relaxation pattern, paying attention to the length and force of the contractions.

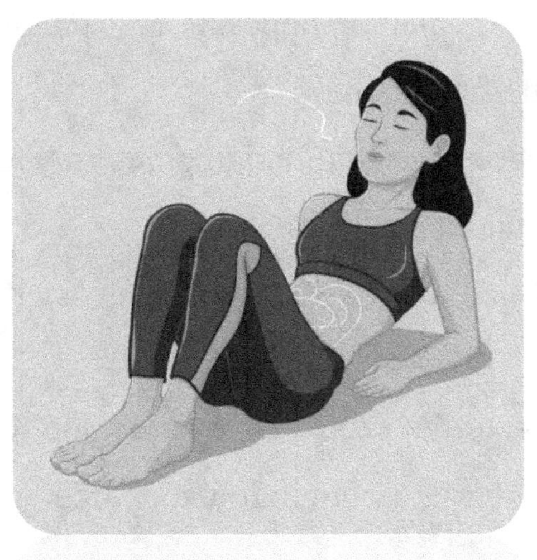

3. Sahrmann Level 1:

1. Begin in a quadruped position on your hands and knees and place your wrists under your shoulders and your knees under your hips.

2. Using your core muscles, raise one arm straight out in front of you and the opposing leg straight back behind you at the same time.

3. After a brief period of holding, return your arm and leg to their initial positions.

4. For a total of 10–12 repetitions, switch sides and repeat on the other side.

5. Throughout the exercise, pay attention to being steady and in control; try not to round or arch your back.

. Sahrmann Level 2:

1. Begin in a quadruped position on your hands and knees and place your wrists under your shoulders and your knees under your hips.

2. Using your core muscles, slowly raise one arm straight out to the side while also raising the opposing leg in the same manner.

3. After a brief period of holding, return your arm and leg to their initial positions.

4. For a total of 10–12 repetitions, switch sides and repeat on the other side.

5. Make sure your pelvis is not twisted or tilted, and maintain your hips level.

5. Seated Marching With Elastic Band:

1. Sit on a chair with your feet flat on the ground and wrap a resistance band around your thighs, slightl above your knees.
2. Lift one foot off the ground and raise your knee up t your chest by using your core muscles.
3. After a brief period of holding, return your foot to th floor and switch to the other side.
4. For a total of 10–12 repetitions, switch up your legs.
5. Pay attention to keeping the resistance band tight an using your hip and core muscles to manage the action.

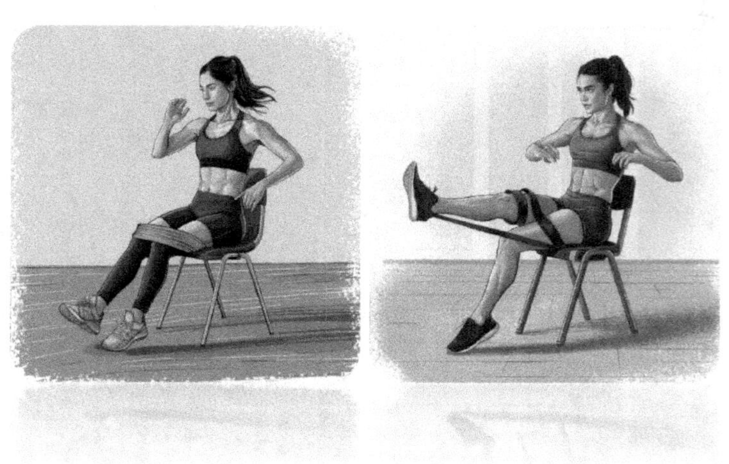

1. Lie on your back, arms at your sides, knees bent, and feet flat on the ground.

2. So that only your heels are touching the ground, raise your toes off the floor.

3. Press through your heels to raise your hips off the ground while using your core muscles.

4. After a few while, maintain the bridge position by lowering your hips back to the floor.

5. Continue for ten to twelve repetitions, keeping your toes raised the entire time to maintain control and stability.

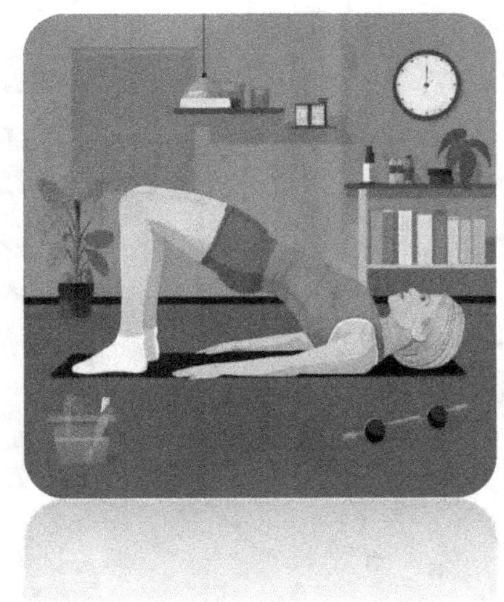

Then lift your toes up

7. Mini Squat:

1. Stand with your toes forward and your feet hip-widt[h]
   apart.

2. As though you were sitting in a chair, carefully lowe[r]
   your body into a squat position by engaging your cor[e]
   muscles.

3. As you descend, keep your knees behind your toes an[d]
   your chest up.

4. After a brief period of holding the squat, push throug[h]
   your heels to get back to the beginning position.

5. Concentrate on correct form and alignment as yo[u]
   perform 10–12 repetitions.

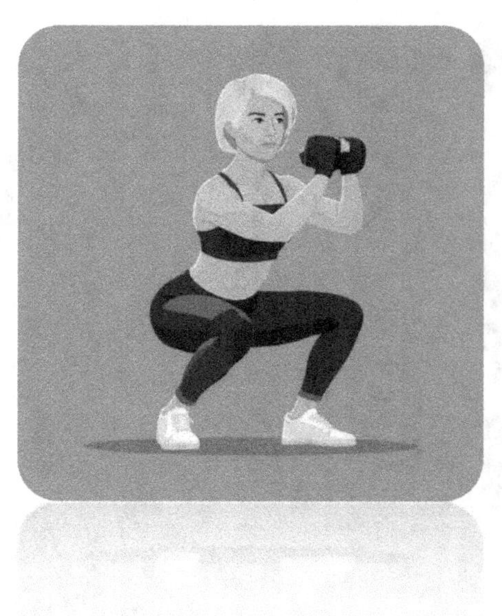

3. Plie Squat:

1. Assume a standing position, spreading your feet wider than hip-width apart and pointing your toes 45 degrees.

2. Maintaining your knees in alignment with your toes, lower your body into a squat by using your core muscles.

3. After a brief period of holding the squat, push through your heels to get back to the beginning position.

4. Ten to twelve repetitions should be performed, with an emphasis on using your pelvic floor and inner thighs.

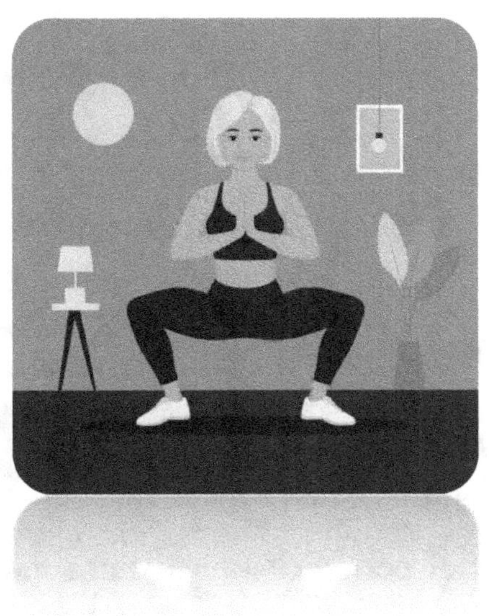

9. Seated Marching with Alternate Arms and Legs:

1. Assume a seated position, placing your hands on your thighs and your feet flat on the ground.

2. As though you were marching in place, raise one foot off the ground and bring the opposing hand up to your shoulder.

3. Repeat on the other side after lowering your raised foot to the ground and hand back.

4. Maintaining stability and synchronization is the major goal as you march for 10 to 12 repetitions on each side, switching up your arms and legs.

10. Standing Marching Single Leg:

1. Your feet should be hip-width apart and keeping your arms loose at your sides.

2. As though you were marching in place, raise one knee towards your chest while maintaining your balance on the other leg.

3. After a brief period of time, return the raised knee to the ground and repeat on the other side.

4. For 10–12 repetitions on each side, keep switching legs in a marching motion while concentrating on balance and stability.

1. Wall Push-Ups:

1. Assume a standing position, face the wall, and extend your arms shoulder-height, pressing your hands flat against the wall.
2. Lower your chest toward the wall by bending your elbows and leaning your body forward while using your core muscles.
3. As you descend, maintain a straight posture from your head to your heels.
4. To straighten your arms and get back to beginning position, push through your palms.
5. Make sure your chest and core muscles are used as you repeat these exercises ten to twelve times.

12. Single-Leg Bridge:

1. Place your feet flat on the floor and lie on your bac
   with your knees bent.
2. Extend one leg straight out in front of you an
   maintaining it parallel to your hip.
3. Press through the heel of your bent leg to raise you
   hips off the ground while using your core muscles.
4. After a few while, maintain the bridge position b
   lowering your hips back to the floor.
5. On each side, perform 8–10 repetitions while keepin
   your balance and control.

13. Single Leg Romanian Deadlift:

1. Assume a tall stance, place your feet hip-width apar
   and keep your arms relaxed by your sides.
2. Put all of your weight on one leg, bend forward at th
   hips, and straighten your other leg behind you.
3. As you drop your torso toward the floor and raise you
   hands to your standing foot, maintain a flat back and
   strong core.

4. To go back to where you started, push through your heel while maintaining a square hip and back.

5. On each side, perform 8–10 repetitions while paying attention to your stability and balance.

4. Bear Crawl:

1. Assume a hands-and-knees position, placing your knees beneath your hips and your wrists beneath your shoulders.

2. Lift your knees off the ground while maintaining a hand-and-toe balance by using your core muscles.

3. Using one hand and the opposing foot simultaneously, crawl forward, and then switch to the other side.

4. For the duration of the designated crawl, keep moving forward while concentrating on remaining stable and under control.

15. Dumbbell Deadlift:

1. Stand tall with your feet hip-width apart, hold dumbbell in each hand, palms facing your thighs an raise yourself up.
2. Maintaining a straight back, descend the dumbbell towards the floor by using your core muscles to lea forward at the hips.
3. As you descend, keep the dumbbells close to you body.
4. To get back to the beginning position, press throug your heels.
5. Continue for 8–10 repetitions with an emphasis o alignment and good form.

Frequently Asked Questions

and Answers

These are frequently asked questions about pelvic floor exercises for women, along with their answers:

1. How frequently should I work out my pelvic floor?

For best effects, try to perform pelvic floor exercises every day. As your muscles grow, progressively increase the duration and intensity of your workouts from three sets of ten to fifteen repetitions every day. Try implementing pelvic floor exercises into your regular routine, like when you brush your teeth or watch TV, as consistency is important.

2. Are there any dangers connected to activities targeting the pelvic floor?

Most women can safely practice pelvic floor exercises when done correctly. But overdoing these workouts or performing them incorrectly might cause tension or tiredness in the muscles. It's crucial to begin with a moderate volume of reps and build up to a higher intensity over time. See a medical expert if you feel any pain or discomfort when performing pelvic floor exercises.

3. Are exercises for the pelvic floor appropriate before, during, and after childbirth?

Exercises targeting the pelvic floor are indeed helpful both during and after pregnancy. Urinary incontinence, pelvic organ prolapse, and other pelvic floor diseases frequently linked to pregnancy and childbirth can be avoided by strengthening the pelvic floor muscles. It's crucial to use the right form and get advice from a medical professional when performing pelvic floor exercises throughout pregnancy and the postpartum period.

4. Can pelvic floor exercises help women going through menopause?

Sure, menopausal women can benefit from pelvic floor exercises to keep their pelvis healthy and to ease problems like dry vagina, diminished libido, and incontinence. By supporting the bladder, uterus, and intestine, strengthening the pelvic floor muscles can enhance pelvic function and quality of life both during and after menopause.

How long do pelvic floor exercises take to show results?

Every person experiences different benefits from pelvic floor exercises, which are contingent on a variety of factors including muscle strength, consistency of training, and adherence to correct technique. After beginning pelvic floor exercises, some women may experience improvements in pelvic support and bladder control in a matter of weeks, while others may require more time to observe noticeable benefits. The secret to getting the results you want is patience and consistent practice.

Is it typical for my pelvic floor muscles to hurt after performing Kegel exercises?

It is common to experience mild discomfort or exhaustion in the pelvic floor muscles, particularly when beginning a new exercise program or increasing the intensity of your workout. On the other hand, excessive exertion or poor technique may be the cause of any acute or ongoing pain. Take breaks as necessary, and seek assessment from a medical expert if discomfort continues.

Yes, some women can benefit from pelvic floor workou
equipment like vaginal weights or biofeedback instruments
especially if they have trouble recognizing or isolating thei
pelvic floor muscles. These gadgets help to activate an
improve muscles by offering resistance and feedback. But it'
imperative that you utilize them appropriately and under
doctor's supervision.

Initially, try to hold each pelvic floor contraction for 5–1(
seconds; as your muscles get stronger, you shoul
progressively extend the holding time. Rather than holding
your breath or tensing other muscles, concentrate on keeping
a continuous and regular contraction. To prevent tiredness
never forget to completely relax your muscles in betweer
contractions.

Exercises targeting the pelvic floor are safe and helpfu
during pregnancy, yes. Enhancing bladder control, promoting

ostpartum recuperation, and supporting the expanding uterus re all made possible by strengthening the pelvic floor muscles. But it is imperative that you exercise caution and efrain from overdoing it. For tailored advice depending on our medical history and stage of pregnancy, speak with your ealthcare practitioner.

0. I've heard about physical treatment for the elvic floor. What is involved, and how may one enefit from it?

A licensed physical therapist with specific training in elvic health will assess and treat patients in pelvic floor hysical therapy. In addition to therapeutic exercises and nformation on the anatomy and function of the pelvic floor, herapy may involve physical techniques and biofeedback. Jumerous pelvic floor issues, such as incontinence, prolapse, elvic discomfort, and sexual dysfunction, can be helped with elvic floor physical therapy.

1. If I've had medical treatments or pelvic urgery, can I still perform pelvic floor xercises?

Yes, pelvic floor exercises can be helpful following nedical treatments or pelvic surgery in many circumstances.

It is imperative that you adhere to any postoperativ
recommendations given by your healthcare professional an
refrain from engaging in any activities that may impede th
healing process. Begin with easy workouts and work you
way up as tolerated, getting your doctor's approval if needed.

12. Should I refrain from doing any particula pelvic floor exercises while I'm pregnant o recovering after giving birth?

While most pelvic floor exercises are acceptable to perforn
during pregnancy and the postpartum period, there are som
high-impact exercises and others that should be avoide
because they put too much strain on the pelvic floor. Intens
abdominal exercises, heavy lifting, and jumping are a few
examples. Pay attention to the low-impact workouts an
pelvic floor strengthening methods that your doctor ha
prescribed.

13. Can someone who has had sexual assault o pelvic trauma perform pelvic floor exercises?

If you have experienced sexual assault or pelvic trauma i
the past, it is imperative that you approach pelvic floo
exercises carefully and sensitively. Certain workouts o
methods might occasionally cause physical or emotiona

distress. Think about consulting with a therapist or healthcare professional who has experience with trauma; they can offer you individualized assistance and direction.

14. How can I keep my pelvic floor healthy over time?

Even after reaching your intended goals, keep doing pelvic floor exercises on a regular basis to preserve pelvic floor health. Include in your workout program movements that focus on posture, total pelvic stability, and core strength. To support pelvic floor function and general well-being, maintain a healthy lifestyle that includes adequate water, a balanced diet, and regular physical activity.

15. Can disorders causing pelvic pain, including vulvodynia or interstitial cystitis, be helped by pelvic floor exercises?

Yes, by increasing pelvic blood flow, lowering muscle tension, and improving muscle tone, pelvic floor exercises may aid in the management of disorders causing pelvic pain. But it's crucial to exercise with caution and collaborate with a medical professional experienced in treating pelvic pain. When combined with other therapies, pelvic floor physical therapy may be helpful in treating pelvic pain in its entirety.

16. Is it typical to have urine leakage when engaging in high-impact exercises like jogging or jumping?

Urinary leakage may occur often during high-impact activities, particularly in women who are undergoing hormonal changes or have just given child. Nonetheless, persistent or substantial leakage could be a symptom of malfunction or weakening in the pelvic floor. Urinary leakage during activities can be managed by using pelvic floor exercises and implementing techniques like wearing protective pads or decreasing the intensity of exercise.

17. Although I've been performing pelvic floor exercises for a few weeks, I haven't seen any results. How should I proceed?

After many weeks of regular pelvic floor training, if you haven't noticed any benefits, think about reevaluating your technique, frequency, and intensity. Make sure your pelvic floor muscles are activated correctly, and increase the intensity of your workouts gradually. Seek examination and individualized coaching from a pelvic floor physical therapist or healthcare provider if progress is still not being made.

88. Can someone with a chronic illness like fibromyalgia or arthritis perform pelvic floor exercises?

Indeed, it is frequently possible to modify pelvic floor exercises for those with long-term medical issues. Prioritizing comfort and safety is crucial, though, and workouts should be adjusted as necessary to account for any restrictions or symptoms. For help creating a customized fitness program that takes into account your unique requirements and concerns, speak with a medical professional or physical therapist who is acquainted with your medical background.

Conclusion

Pelvic floor exercises, also known as Kegel exercises, are a fundamental component of women's health. They are essential in preventing diseases like pelvic organ prolapse and urine incontinence by fortifying the muscles that support the uterus, bladder, and bowels.

Women who are pregnant or who have recently given birth can benefit most from these exercises because these life events can put a great deal of strain on the pelvic muscles. Frequent pelvic floor training can aid in the recovery of these muscles and lower the likelihood of problems after childbirth.

Furthermore, it has been discovered that pelvic floor exercises enhance sexual pleasure and health, which makes them advantageous for women of all ages. They can also help in the healing process following gynecological procedures like hysterectomy.

Though they have many advantages, pelvic floor exercises require proper execution to yield desired results. Inadequate execution may result in minimal progress or worsen pre existing issues.

It is therefore advised to learn these exercises from a licensed healthcare provider, such as a physiotherapist with a focus on women's health.

Moreover, when it comes to pelvic floor exercises, consistency is essential.

To keep the pelvic muscles strong, they must be performed consistently over an extended length of time. It requires a sustained commitment to one's health rather than a short fix.

Finally, even though pelvic floor exercises are quite helpful, they cannot treat every pelvic health problem on their own.

They ought to be a part of an all-encompassing strategy for women's health that also consists of frequent examinations, a healthy diet, and an active way of life.

Essentially, pelvic floor exercises are an easy-to-use yet effective practice that can help women's health.

They serve as evidence that sometimes the simplest things can have the biggest positive effects on one's health.

Bonus Pages

1. Quinoa and Vegetable Buddha Bowl:

Ingredients:

1 cup of quinoa

2 cups of mixed veggies (carrots, broccoli, and bell peppers)

1 sliced avocado

A handful of halved cherry tomatoes

¼ cup of hummus

Slices of lemon.

Fresh chopped herbs (parsley, cilantro, etc.)

Instructions:

1. Prepare the quinoa as directed on the package and set aside.

2. Sauté mixed vegetables in a skillet until tender.

3. Put cooked quinoa, cherry tomatoes, sautéed veggies, avocado slices, and a dollop of hummus in bowls.

4. Add chopped herbs as a garnish and squeeze fresh lemon juice over the bowls.

5. Savor as a filling meal that supports pelvic floor health with necessary minerals, fiber, and protein.

2. Turkey and Vegetables Stir-Fry:

Ingredients:

1 pound, lean ground turkey

2 cups of mixed vegetables, like carrots, snap peas, and bell peppers

2 tsps. Of soy sauce with low sodium

1 tsp. of sesame oil

2 minced garlic cloves

1 tsp. finely grated ginger

Ready-to-serve cooked brown rice

Optional garnish of sesame seeds

Instructions:

1. In a large skillet or wok over medium-high heat, heat the sesame oil.

. Add the ground turkey to the skillet and sauté it until it is thoroughly cooked and browned.

. Cook for a further minute or until aromatic after adding the minced garlic and grated ginger to the skillet.

. Add the mixed vegetables to the skillet and cook, stirring, until they become tender.

. Cook for a further two to three minutes after stirring in low-sodium soy sauce.

. Spoon cooked brown rice over the turkey and vegetable stir-fry.

. Add sesame seeds as a garnish if you'd like, then savor your tasty and high-protein dinner.

3. Mediterranean Chickpea Salad:

Ingredients:

can (15 Oz) of rinsed and drained chickpeas

diced cucumber

1 cup of halved cherry tomatoes

1/4 cup of finely chopped red onion

1/4 cup of sliced Kalamata olives

2 tsp. of chopped fresh parsley

2 tsp. extra virgin olive oil

1 tsp. of lemon juice

1 tsp. of dried oregano

Add salt and pepper to taste.

Instructions:

1. Put the chickpeas, cucumber, cherry tomatoes, red onion, Kalamata olives, and fresh parsley in a big bowl.

2. In a small bowl, whisk together extra virgin olive oil, lemon juice, dried oregano, salt, and pepper to make the dressing.

3. After pouring the dressing over the salad, gently toss to coat.

. To let the flavors combine, refrigerate for a minimum of alf an hour.

. Present chilled as a wholesome and revitalizing dish that is bundant in fiber, protein, and healthy fats.

. Vegetable and Lentil Soup:

ngredients:

tsp. of olive oil

chopped onion

chopped carrots

diced celery stalks

minced garlic cloves

cup of washed and dried green lentils

cups of vegetable broth

can of diced tomatoes (14 oz.)

cups of chopped of spinach or greens

1 tsp. of dried thyme

Add salt and pepper to taste.

Instructions:

1. In a big saucepan, warm up the olive oil over medium heat. Add the diced onion, celery, and carrots and sauté until the veggies are tender.

2. Add the minced garlic and sauté for a further minute until fragrant.

3. Add the chopped tomatoes, dried thyme, vegetable broth, and dried green lentils. Heat up until boiling.

4. Lower the heat to a simmer, cover, and let the lentils cook for 25 to 30 minutes, or until they are soft.

5. During the last five minutes of simmering, add chopped spinach or kale to the soup.

6. Toss in some pepper and salt, to taste.

Serve hot for a filling, nourishing meal that's high in fiber, vitamins, and minerals.

5. Greek Yogurt Parfait with Berry and Almonds:

Ingredients:

1 cup of Greek yogurt

½ cup of mixed berries, including blueberries, raspberries, and strawberries

2 tsp. Of chopped Almonds

1 tsp. of optional honey

¼ tsp. of vanilla extract

Instructions:

1. Gently stir together the Greek yogurt, honey (if desired), and vanilla extract in a small bowl.

2. In a glass or bowl, layer Greek yogurt, sliced almonds, and a mixture of berries.

3. Continue layering until all ingredients have been utilized. Top with a final sprinkle of almond slices.

4. Serve right away as a tasty and wholesome dessert or snack that is high in fiber, protein, and vital vitamins and minerals.

www.ingramcontent.com/pod-product-compliance
Lightning Source LLC
Chambersburg PA
CBHW050819250726

48653CB00006B/2310